Motivational Interviewing for Pharmacists

A Practical Guide to Medication Adherence Conversations, Patient Counseling Scripts, and Behavior Change at the Counter

Honor Victoria Frost

Copyright and Disclaimer

First Edition

ISBN; 979-8-90678-200-7

Staten House

Table of Contents

Preface

Medication adherence remains one of the most persistent challenges in contemporary pharmacy practice. Large-scale analyses continue to document substantial clinical and economic consequences of nonoptimized medication therapy, yet the daily conversations that could influence patient behavior often default to rapid information delivery. Time pressure, limited formal communication training, and the natural tendency to correct or persuade combine to produce encounters that frequently leave both pharmacist and patient frustrated.

Motivational interviewing is a collaborative, goal-oriented style of communication that strengthens a person's own motivation for change by exploring their reasons within an atmosphere of acceptance and partnership (Miller & Rollnick, 2013). It is distinct from standard patient education, persuasive counseling, and nondirective listening. Where traditional approaches prioritize the transfer of clinical facts, motivational interviewing prioritizes the patient's language of change and the relational conditions that allow that language to emerge.

Most pharmacists and pharmacy technicians receive little sustained preparation in these methods. Concepts may appear briefly in curricula or continuing education, yet the translation into the two-to-five-minute realities of the counter or clinic remains incomplete. The result is a gap between knowing that collaborative conversations matter and possessing usable words, structure, and habits that survive ordinary workflow demands.

This book addresses that gap directly. It presents the spirit of motivational interviewing, the core OARS micro-skills, a compressed conversation structure suited to pharmacy time, ready scripts for common adherence situations, and guidance for involving technicians and students. Realistic examples and process measures support application rather than abstract understanding. The aim is practical competence: the ability to conduct brief, respectful conversations that reduce unnecessary resistance and invite patients to articulate their own reasons for change.

The primary readers are community and clinical pharmacists, pharmacy technicians, and PharmD students who counsel patients regularly. Secondary readers include preceptors, pharmacy managers, and educators seeking shared language for team training. The book does not replace formal clinical decision-making, comprehensive medication management services, or organization-specific protocols. It offers no assurance of specific adherence rates or clinical outcomes. It supplies a structured method for improving the quality of everyday counseling conversations under real constraints.

The purpose of the following chapters is to equip readers with clear, usable skills for brief motivational interviewing at the pharmacy counter.

Chapter 1.0: Nonadherence Costs and Limits

The estimated annual cost of prescription drug-related morbidity and mortality from nonoptimized medication therapy stood at $528.4 billion in 2016 U.S. dollars (Watanabe et al., 2018). That figure, drawn from nationally representative data and modeling of treatment failures and new medical problems, equals roughly 16 percent of total U.S. health care expenditures for the year. The plausible range ran from $495.3 billion to $672.7 billion. The average cost pathway for one patient experiencing treatment failure, a new medical problem, or both after an initial prescription hovered near $2,500. These numbers raise a direct question for every pharmacist who counsels at the counter or in clinic: if the downstream harm is this large, why do so many brief conversations still end with patients walking away no more likely to take the medicine as prescribed?

1.1 Scale of the Problem

Nonoptimized medication therapy includes more than simple forgetfulness. It covers unfilled prescriptions, incorrect doses, early discontinuation, and regimens that create new problems while failing to resolve the original ones. Watanabe and colleagues modeled these pathways using federal data sources, nursing home surveys, and validated cost estimates inflated to 2016 dollars (Watanabe et al., 2018). Their work updated earlier figures that had placed the burden near $290 billion in 2008. The jump reflects both rising medical costs and persistent gaps between prescribed therapy and actual patient behavior.

Pharmacists see the human side of those numbers every shift. A patient with hypertension refills late or not at all. Blood pressure climbs. An emergency department visit follows. A statin sits in the bottle because the patient felt fine and saw no immediate need. Cholesterol rises. A cardiac event occurs months later.

Each individual story is modest. Multiplied across hundreds of millions of prescriptions, the aggregate becomes the half-trillion-dollar figure.

Community pharmacists occupy a uniquely frequent contact point. More than 90 percent of Americans live within five miles of a community pharmacy (Kelling, 2015). Refill visits, new prescription counseling, and medication therapy management encounters create repeated opportunities to influence adherence. Yet time pressure, high volume, and habitual counseling styles often convert those opportunities into rapid information dumps that patients neither retain nor act upon. The economic data make the missed chance expensive for the system. The daily experience makes it costly for the pharmacist who wants better outcomes and leaves the encounter frustrated.

1.2 Why Information Alone Fails

Traditional counseling rests on a reasonable but incomplete assumption: if patients understand the benefits and risks, they will choose the recommended action. Pharmacists therefore explain mechanism, dosing, side effects, and monitoring. The patient nods. The pharmacist documents counseling. The prescription leaves the counter. Weeks later the refill is late or absent.

The assumption breaks down because most patients already possess partial information and still remain ambivalent. Ambivalence is the simultaneous presence of reasons for and against change. A patient may accept that high blood pressure raises stroke risk while also believing the medicine will make them feel worse or signal that they are "really sick." Information that addresses only one side of the ambivalence leaves the other side untouched and often strengthens it. When a pharmacist pushes harder with more facts, the patient frequently defends the status quo more vigorously. Researchers describe this as the righting reflex: the clinician's urge to correct, persuade, or fix

(Miller & Rollnick, 2013). The reflex is well intentioned. It is also predictably counterproductive.

Miller and Rollnick developed motivational interviewing precisely to address this pattern. Their definition frames the method as a collaborative, goal-oriented style of communication that pays particular attention to the language of change. It strengthens personal motivation by eliciting and exploring the person's own reasons for change within an atmosphere of acceptance and compassion (Miller & Rollnick, 2013). The method originated in addiction treatment (Miller, 1983) and later spread across health care because the same ambivalence appears in medication taking, smoking cessation, diet change, and vaccine decisions.

Berger and Villaume adapted the approach specifically for health care professionals, including pharmacists (Berger & Villaume, 2013). Their work emphasizes sense-making: patients continuously interpret their symptoms, diagnoses, and treatments. Effective counseling first reflects that sense-making accurately and nonjudgmentally, then offers missing or corrective information in a form the patient can integrate without losing face. The sequence reduces relational resistance and opens space for the patient to reconsider.

1.3 Everyday Barriers at the Counter

Time remains the most frequently cited obstacle. Qualitative studies of community pharmacists repeatedly surface the "fight for time" (Jalal et al., 2019). Dispensing targets, waiting customers, and concurrent clinical tasks compress counseling into two or three minutes. In that window the default script is efficient information delivery. Reflection, open questions, and exploration of ambivalence feel like luxuries the schedule cannot afford.

A second barrier is anticipated negative reaction. Pharmacists report hesitating to raise nonadherence because they expect defensiveness, argument, or complaint. The expectation is not baseless. Traditional confrontational or heavily persuasive styles do provoke resistance. The anticipation itself, however, reduces the number of conversations attempted.

Training gaps compound the problem. Many PharmD curricula introduce motivational interviewing as an elective or brief module. Students learn the acronyms but receive limited supervised practice under realistic time pressure. Graduates enter practice knowing the concepts yet defaulting to the styles they observed during rotations. Continuing education courses exist, yet uptake is uneven and skills decay without deliberate reinforcement.

Privacy and workflow design create further friction. Open counseling areas limit depth. Interruptions fracture attention. Electronic systems prompt counseling documentation but rarely support the conversational structure that would make the documentation meaningful.

These barriers are real. They do not, however, make brief, effective conversations impossible. Micro-adaptations of motivational interviewing skills fit inside existing time windows. The remainder of this book develops those adaptations. First it is necessary to see clearly what the current pattern costs and why it persists.

1.4 A Composite Case of Missed Opportunity

Consider a composite case built from common pharmacy patterns. Arden, a 58-year-old patient with type 2 diabetes and hypertension, arrives for refills of metformin and lisinopril. The dispensing record shows both prescriptions are 18 days late. The pharmacist, Bellamy, recognizes the gap and opens the conversation with a standard counseling script.

"Arden, your blood sugar and blood pressure medicines are important. Missing doses can raise your risk of kidney problems and heart attack. You should take them every day as prescribed. Do you have any questions about side effects or how to take them?"

Arden replies, "I feel fine most of the time. The metformin upsets my stomach if I don't eat enough. I'll try to be better."

Bellamy adds a few more points about consistent timing and food, documents the counseling, and moves to the next patient. Three months later both prescriptions are again late. A1C has risen. Blood pressure readings in the pharmacy kiosk are higher than previous visits.

The exchange contained accurate clinical information. It also followed the classic righting-reflex pattern: the clinician stated the problem and the solution, then checked for questions. Arden's ambivalence about stomach upset and the sense that feeling fine reduced urgency never received reflection or exploration. The conversation ended with a polite commitment that carried little behavioral weight.

A different sequence, still completed in under four minutes, might have begun with an open question and a reflection: "I notice the refills are a bit behind. What's been getting in the way of taking them regularly?" After listening, a simple reflection of the stomach concern and the "feeling fine" belief, followed by permission to share one piece of information about asymptomatic progression, would have invited Arden to weigh the trade-offs rather than defend against advice. The outcome is not guaranteed. The process, however, aligns with the evidence on how motivation actually shifts.

1.5 What the Evidence Shows About Brief Interventions

Studies of pharmacist-delivered motivational interviewing, even when brief, show measurable effects on adherence and related clinical markers. Telephone-based interventions by pharmacists or pharmacy students trained in the method have improved proportion of days covered for antihypertensives, antihyperlipidemics, and antidiabetics (Abughosh et al., 2017). Medicare Star Ratings in some plans moved upward after structured motivational interviewing programs were implemented (Spears et al., 2020). Vaccine acceptance conversations that use open questions, reflections, and autonomy support rather than persuasion increase uptake in hesitant patients (Gagneur, 2020).

The effect sizes are moderate rather than dramatic. That is consistent with the nature of behavior change. A single three-minute conversation rarely transforms a lifelong pattern. Repeated, skillful conversations accumulate. They also preserve the relationship so that future conversations remain possible. In contrast, repeated righting-reflex encounters can erode trust and make later attempts more difficult.

The economic modeling by Watanabe and colleagues points toward comprehensive medication management as one scalable response (Watanabe et al., 2018). Motivational interviewing skills form a practical core of that management when delivered at the point of dispensing or during scheduled clinical services. The skills do not require a private office or a 30-minute appointment. They require a shift in conversational posture and a small set of practiced micro-skills.

1.6 The Righting Reflex in Daily Practice

Every pharmacist has felt the urge to correct. A patient states an inaccurate belief about a medicine. The clinician's knowledge lights up. Words form that will set the record straight. The patient then pushes back or shuts down. The cycle is so common that many practitioners stop noticing it.

The reflex is not a character flaw. It arises from genuine concern and from professional training that emphasizes accurate information. Motivational interviewing does not ask pharmacists to abandon expertise. It asks them to place that expertise in the service of the patient's own emerging motivation rather than in opposition to the patient's current position. The practical difference appears in sequence and tone. First understand and reflect. Then, with permission, offer information that addresses the specific concern the patient has voiced. Finally, ask the patient what sense they make of the new information.

This sequence respects autonomy. It also increases the chance that the patient will voice change talk (statements that favor the desired behavior) rather than sustain talk (statements that favor the status quo). Change talk predicts subsequent behavior change more reliably than clinician advice (Amrhein et al., 2003).

1.7 Bridging to Practical Skills

The cost data and the conversational patterns described here set the stage for the skills that follow. Later chapters detail the spirit of motivational interviewing, the OARS micro-skills, the structure of a two-to-five-minute conversation, ready scripts for common pharmacy situations, and adaptations for high-stakes topics such as vaccine hesitancy and new injectable therapies. Each chapter keeps the time constraint and the counter environment in view.

The $528.4 billion figure is not an abstract policy number. It is the cumulative result of millions of individual decisions made, deferred, or reversed after brief encounters with pharmacists and other clinicians. Improving the quality of those encounters will not erase the entire burden. It will, however, move a measurable portion of it in the right direction while restoring a sense of professional effectiveness to the people who stand at the counter every day.

Essential Takeaways

The scale of nonoptimized medication therapy reaches hundreds of billions of dollars each year and touches nearly every chronic disease the pharmacy sees. Traditional information-heavy counseling frequently fails because it collides with patient ambivalence and activates the righting reflex. Pharmacists already occupy the contact points where brief, skilled conversations can influence those decisions. Time pressure and training gaps are real obstacles, yet they do not preclude micro-adaptations of motivational interviewing. A single composite case of late refills illustrates how the same clinical facts can be delivered in a way that either invites or suppresses patient engagement. Evidence from pharmacist-delivered interventions supports the value of even short encounters that prioritize partnership and the patient's own language of change. The next chapters turn from diagnosis of the problem to the concrete skills that address it.

Chapter 2.0: Spirit of Motivational Interviewing

The pharmacy counter is crowded. A technician calls the next number. Briar steps forward holding a white paper bag and a half-empty water bottle. The pharmacist, Calloway, glances at the profile: new start on a GLP-1 receptor agonist, prior metformin, recent A1C of 8.4. Calloway begins the usual counseling points about injection technique, gastrointestinal side effects, and the need for gradual dose titration. Briar interrupts after the second sentence. "I already looked it up. I'm worried it will make me sick every day and I won't be able to work. Maybe I'll just try harder with diet." Calloway feels the familiar pull to correct the concern with more data on efficacy and tolerability rates. The next patient is already waiting.

2.1 Opening the Case Without Theory

Briar's statement contains both sustain talk and a hint of change talk. The fear of daily nausea is real and grounded in common experience with the class. The mention of trying harder with diet shows residual motivation for glycemic control. Traditional counseling would meet the fear with reassurance statistics and then pivot back to the prescribed plan. That sequence often leaves the patient defending the fear more strongly. The conversation ends with a polite nod and low likelihood of follow-through.

In this chapter the same encounter is examined through the lens of the underlying spirit of motivational interviewing rather than through techniques first. The spirit is the set of relational attitudes that make the later skills effective. Without it the skills become mechanical and can feel manipulative. With it the briefest exchange can shift from confrontation to collaboration.

2.2 Partnership Instead of Expert Authority

Partnership treats the patient as the expert on their own life, values, and constraints while the pharmacist remains the expert on the medication. The two forms of expertise are complementary, not hierarchical. In the opening scene Calloway holds the clinical knowledge about the GLP-1 agent. Briar holds the knowledge about work schedules, prior side-effect experiences, and personal tolerance for discomfort. A partnership stance begins by acknowledging both sources of knowledge rather than overriding one with the other.

Miller and Rollnick describe partnership as an active collaboration in which the clinician avoids the expert trap of assuming responsibility for the patient's decisions (Miller & Rollnick, 2013). Berger and Villaume, writing for health care professionals, emphasize that patients continuously make sense of their conditions and treatments (Berger & Villaume, 2013). The pharmacist's first task is to understand that sense-making accurately before offering new information. When Calloway responds to Briar with "You're concerned the side effects could interfere with work, and you're weighing whether diet changes might be enough," the reflection signals that Briar's perspective has been heard. Only after that recognition does new information have a chance of being considered rather than resisted.

Partnership does not mean the pharmacist withholds expertise. It means the expertise is offered inside a relationship that already respects the patient's autonomy. The practical difference appears in the order of talk. Reflection and exploration come before advice. Permission is requested before information is delivered. The patient is invited to interpret the new information rather than simply receive it.

2.3 Acceptance of the Person and the Ambivalence

Acceptance in motivational interviewing has four interlocking elements: absolute worth, accurate empathy, autonomy support, and affirmation (Miller & Rollnick, 2013). Absolute worth means the patient is treated as inherently valuable regardless of current behavior. Accurate empathy means the clinician seeks to understand the patient's internal frame without judgment. Autonomy support means the right to choose, including the right not to change, is explicitly honored. Affirmation means genuine strengths and efforts are noticed and named.

In Briar's case, acceptance looks like this: the pharmacist does not argue that the fear of nausea is exaggerated. Instead the fear is treated as understandable given the patient's work demands. The desire to manage diabetes through diet is affirmed as evidence of caring about health. The autonomy to decide whether to start the injection is left with Briar. This stance reduces defensiveness. Patients who feel accepted are more willing to examine their own ambivalence rather than defend against external pressure.

Acceptance is frequently misunderstood as passive agreement. It is not. A pharmacist can fully accept a patient's current position and still hold a clear clinical opinion about the better long-term path. The acceptance is of the person and of the reality of ambivalence, not of the clinical conclusion. When the patient experiences that acceptance, the psychological need to protect the status quo diminishes and space opens for reconsideration.

2.4 Compassion as Priority of the Other's Welfare

Compassion is the deliberate commitment to pursue the welfare and best interests of the patient (Miller & Rollnick, 2013). It is distinguished from sympathy or pity. In the pharmacy setting it appears as genuine concern for how the medication regimen will fit the patient's actual life rather than an abstract ideal life. For Briar, compassion means taking the work-related nausea concern seriously rather than dismissing it as secondary to the A1C number.

Compassion also protects the pharmacist from the burnout that comes with repeated unsuccessful persuasion. When the clinician's self-worth is tied to whether the patient complies, every nonadherent refill feels like personal failure. When the clinician's commitment is to the patient's welfare as the patient defines it, the conversation remains purposeful even when the immediate outcome is not full adherence. The pharmacist has still offered a respectful, skillful opportunity for change.

2.5 Evocation of the Patient's Own Motivation

Evocation is the opposite of installation. Instead of installing motivation from the outside, the clinician draws out the motivation already present within the patient (Miller & Rollnick, 2013). Most patients who reach the pharmacy counter already possess reasons for better health. Those reasons may be temporarily overshadowed by fears, logistics, or competing priorities. The clinician's task is to help the patient hear their own reasons more clearly.

In the opening scene, Briar has already voiced a desire to manage diabetes. The diet comment is change talk, even if partial. An evocative response would explore that desire further: "You mentioned trying harder with diet. What matters to you about keeping your blood sugar in a better range?" The question invites Briar to articulate personal values rather than respond to the pharmacist's values. Once those values are spoken aloud by the patient, they carry more motivational weight than any statistic the pharmacist could provide.

Evocation requires curiosity and restraint. The pharmacist must resist the urge to fill silence with advice and must listen for the patient's language of change. When that language appears, the clinician reflects it, strengthens it, and asks the patient to elaborate. The result is that the patient, not the clinician, becomes the primary source of arguments for change.

2.6 A Second Case of Spirit in Action

A composite case from community practice illustrates the difference the spirit makes under time pressure. Dune, a 64-year-old patient, picks up a new prescription for atorvastatin after a recent lipid panel. The pharmacist, Ellis, has ninety seconds before the next patient. Dune says, "My brother took one of these and had muscle pain. I'm not sure I want to start."

An expert-authority response would list the low incidence of myopathy, the benefits of LDL reduction, and the monitoring plan. An acceptance-and-evocation response begins differently: "You're cautious because of what happened with your brother, and you want to protect yourself from the same problem." After a brief pause, "What do you already know about the muscle side effect, and what would help you feel safer if you decided to try it?" The reflection and open question take less than thirty seconds. They communicate acceptance of the concern and invite Dune to participate in solving it. Ellis can then, with permission, provide the incidence data and the recommendation to report any unexplained muscle symptoms promptly. The conversation remains brief. The relational tone is different. Dune leaves having been heard rather than persuaded.

2.7 Common Misreadings of the Spirit

Three frequent misunderstandings undermine the spirit in pharmacy practice. The first is that partnership means the pharmacist has no opinion. Partnership means the opinion is offered collaboratively, not that it is abandoned. The second is that acceptance requires the pharmacist to agree with nonadherence. Acceptance is of the person and the ambivalence, not of the clinical outcome. The third is that evocation is passive. Evocation is active, strategic listening and questioning aimed at drawing out the patient's own change language.

When these misunderstandings take hold, pharmacists either abandon the approach as too soft or apply the techniques without the underlying attitudes. Both results are ineffective. The spirit is not optional packaging. It is the operating system that makes the later skills coherent and ethical.

2.8 Linking Spirit to the Counter Reality

The spirit must survive contact with the actual pharmacy environment. High volume, interruptions, and performance metrics do not disappear. The claim of this chapter is not that pharmacists can conduct leisurely counseling sessions. The claim is that the same two-to-five-minute window can be used in a way that either activates or reduces patient defensiveness. The spirit guides the choice of words and the sequence of talk inside that window.

Later chapters translate the spirit into concrete micro-skills and scripts. Those tools only work when the relational stance described here is present. Without partnership, acceptance, compassion, and evocation, the skills become another form of persuasion. With them, the briefest exchange can leave the patient more, rather than less, open to change.

The Practitioner's Takeaways

The opening encounter with Briar shows how quickly the righting reflex can appear and how readily a different stance can change the tone. Partnership recognizes two experts in the conversation. Acceptance reduces the need for the patient to defend. Compassion keeps the focus on the patient's welfare as the patient experiences it. Evocation draws motivation from inside the patient rather than installing it from outside. These four elements form the spirit that makes motivational interviewing coherent. A second brief case with Dune demonstrates that the spirit can be enacted in under two minutes. Common misreadings that treat the spirit as passive or opinionfree are corrected by returning to the original definitions. The practical implication for the busy pharmacist is straightforward: the attitude you bring to the first ten seconds of the conversation largely determines whether the remaining seconds will be spent in collaboration or in quiet resistance. The skills that follow in later chapters rest on this foundation.

Chapter 3.0: Core OARS Micro Skills

You stand at the counseling window with a patient who has just said, "I know I should take it, but I keep forgetting." Your next sentence will either open the conversation or close it. Most pharmacists reach for a reminder strategy or a warning about consequences. The OARS skills give you four other moves that take the same amount of time and produce a different result.

3.1 Why Micro Skills Matter Under Time Pressure

OARS stands for open questions, affirmations, reflections, and summaries (Miller & Rollnick, 2013). These are the technical skills that put the spirit of motivational interviewing into words. They are deliberately simple so they can be used in the two-to-five-minute windows that define community and clinic pharmacy practice. When the skills are absent, even a well-intentioned pharmacist defaults to closed questions, unsolicited advice, and the righting reflex. When the skills are present, the same short encounter can elicit change talk and reduce resistance.

The skills are not a rigid sequence. They are a set of options the pharmacist selects in real time according to what the patient has just said. Mastery comes from deliberate practice of each skill in isolation and then in combination. This chapter treats them as operational tools rather than abstract theory.

3.2 Open Questions That Fit the Counter

An open question is one that cannot be answered with a single word or a simple yes or no. It invites the patient to talk. In a busy pharmacy the goal is not a long narrative. The goal is a response long enough to reveal the patient's current thinking so the pharmacist can respond accurately.

Useful open questions in pharmacy settings are short and focused. "What has been getting in the way of taking it regularly?" "How are you feeling about starting this one?" "What do you already know about the side effects?" Each question can be spoken in under three seconds and still yields usable information.

Closed questions remain appropriate for safety checks and confirmation. "Have you ever had trouble swallowing pills?" is efficient and necessary. The error occurs when closed questions dominate the entire counseling encounter. A string of closed questions turns the patient into a passive respondent and the pharmacist into an interrogator. One or two well-chosen open questions early in the exchange change the dynamic.

A common confusion is the belief that open questions must be elaborate. They do not. The simplest open questions are often the most effective under time pressure. "What's your sense of this?" or "How does that sound to you?" keep the floor with the patient without requiring a lengthy reply.

3.3 Affirmations That Feel Genuine

An affirmation notices and names a strength, effort, or positive quality in the patient. It is distinct from praise. Praise evaluates ("Good job"). Affirmation recognizes ("You have been consistent with the metformin for three months"). The grammatical difference is small. The relational difference is large. Praise positions the pharmacist as the judge. Affirmation positions the pharmacist as a witness to the patient's own capabilities.

Effective affirmations in pharmacy are specific and accurate. "You made it in today even though the weather is bad" is concrete. "You're really dedicated to your health" is vague and can feel hollow. Patients detect inauthenticity quickly. When the affirmation matches something the patient has actually done or said, it builds confidence and rapport in a few words.

Affirmations are underused because pharmacists fear sounding soft or wasting time. In practice a single accurate affirmation takes two seconds and often produces a visible shift in the patient's posture or tone. It also models the nonjudgmental stance that makes later information easier to receive.

3.4 Reflections as the Primary Tool

Reflective listening is the core skill of motivational interviewing (Miller & Rollnick, 2013). A reflection is a statement that returns the patient's meaning to them, usually in slightly different words. It serves three purposes at once: it demonstrates that the pharmacist has heard accurately, it allows the patient to hear their own thoughts more clearly, and it encourages further elaboration without a new question.

Simple reflections stay close to the patient's words. Patient: "The pills make me feel tired." Pharmacist: "The tiredness is bothering you." Complex reflections add inferred meaning or emotional content. "The tiredness is getting in the way of your day, and you're wondering whether it's worth it." Both forms are useful. Simple reflections are safer when the pharmacist is still learning. Complex reflections, when accurate, deepen the conversation faster.

Reflections are the most efficient way to handle resistance. When a patient voices sustain talk, a reflection of that talk often reduces its intensity. Arguing with it increases its intensity. The pharmacist does not have to agree with the content. The pharmacist only has to show that the content has been understood.

Under time pressure the temptation is to skip reflection and move straight to advice. The cost of that skip is frequently a defensive patient and a wasted counseling moment. A single accurate reflection costs almost no time and often saves the rest of the encounter from becoming an argument.

3.5 Summaries That Close or Transition

A summary is a collection of reflections that pulls together what the patient has said. In a brief pharmacy encounter the summary is usually short: two or three sentences that capture the key points the patient has voiced. It can be used to close the conversation, to transition to information giving, or to check that the pharmacist has understood correctly.

A well-built summary often includes both sides of the patient's ambivalence when both have been expressed. "So on one hand you're concerned about the stomach upset, and on the other hand you want to get the A1C down so you can stay active with your grandkids." The patient hears the full picture and is invited to resolve it. The pharmacist has not taken sides.

Summaries also serve a practical documentation function. The act of summarizing forces the pharmacist to notice what actually mattered to the patient, which improves the quality of any note that follows.

3.6 Combining the Skills in Real Time

The four skills are rarely used in isolation. A typical brief sequence might look like this: open question, reflection of the answer, affirmation of effort, another reflection or open question, then a short summary that leads to permission to share information. The entire sequence can fit inside three minutes.

The order is not fixed. If the patient opens with strong sustain talk, the pharmacist may begin with a reflection rather than a question. If the patient has already shown clear effort, an affirmation may be the first move. The guiding principle is responsiveness to what the patient has just offered rather than adherence to a memorized script.

Practice begins with single skills. A pharmacist can decide, for one shift, to use at least three accurate reflections. On the next shift the focus can shift to open questions. Over time the skills become automatic and can be selected fluidly.

3.7 Worked Example with Fallon

Fallon, a 47-year-old patient, presents a new prescription for an antidepressant. The profile shows a previous trial that was discontinued after two weeks. The pharmacist, Garnet, has limited time.

Fallon: "I tried one of these before and it made me feel worse at first. I'm not sure I want to go through that again."

Garnet (reflection): "The early side effects last time left you hesitant to start another one."

Fallon: "Yeah. I felt more anxious for about ten days and almost stopped."

Garnet (open question): "What helped you get through those first days last time, or what made you stop?"

Fallon: "I stopped. I didn't know it might get better."

Garnet (affirmation): "You paid close attention to how you were feeling and made a decision based on that."

Fallon: "I guess."

Garnet (summary and permission): "So the last experience started rough and you didn't have information that the early increase in anxiety can settle. Would it be all right if I shared what usually happens in the first two weeks with this medicine and how we monitor it?"

The exchange remains brief. Fallon has been heard, an accurate strength has been named, and information is now offered with permission rather than imposed. The OARS skills structured the entire conversation.

3.8 Common Errors and Corrections

Three errors appear repeatedly when pharmacists first practice OARS. The first is the interrogating style: a rapid series of open questions without reflections in between. The patient feels questioned rather than understood. The correction is to follow most questions with a reflection of the answer before asking another question.

The second error is the fake affirmation. Generic statements such as "You're doing great" that do not match anything specific the patient has done. Patients discount them. The correction is to affirm only what is observable or what the patient has explicitly stated.

The third error is the complex reflection that misses the mark. When the inferred meaning is wrong, the patient corrects it, which is useful, but repeated misses erode confidence. The correction is to stay closer to the patient's words until accuracy improves.

These errors are normal in the learning phase. They diminish with deliberate practice and feedback.

Putting It to Work

Open questions invite the patient's perspective without requiring lengthy answers. Affirmations notice real strengths and build confidence in seconds. Reflections demonstrate understanding, reduce resistance, and keep the conversation collaborative. Summaries gather the threads and create clean transitions to information or closure. The four skills are operational tools designed for the time constraints of pharmacy practice. A single worked encounter with Fallon shows how they combine into a coherent brief conversation. Common early errors are correctable through focused practice of one skill at a time. The next chapter places these micro skills inside a repeatable structure that fits the two-to-five-minute counter window.

Chapter 4.0: Brief Conversation Structure

The same three minutes can be used in two completely different ways. One way leaves the patient nodding and unlikely to change. The other leaves the patient having voiced a reason for change that belongs to them. The difference is structure.

4.1 The Problem of Unstructured Counseling

Most pharmacy counseling follows an implicit script shaped by regulation and habit: verify identity, state the name and purpose of the medicine, cover directions and warnings, ask if there are questions, document. The script is efficient for information transfer. It is poorly suited to behavior change. It places the pharmacist in the directing role from the first sentence and leaves little room for the patient's own motivation to surface.

When time is short the unstructured or purely informational approach feels safest. The cost is repeated encounters that produce little lasting effect on adherence. A minimal structure that still respects the clock can change the outcome without lengthening the encounter.

4.2 Four Processes Adapted to Pharmacy Time

Miller and Rollnick describe four overlapping processes in motivational interviewing: engaging, focusing, evoking, and planning (Miller & Rollnick, 2013). In a twenty-minute counseling session the processes can unfold with room to breathe. In a pharmacy counter encounter they must be compressed. The compression is possible when the pharmacist knows which process is needed at each moment.

Engaging is the establishment of a working relationship. At the counter it often takes one accurate reflection or one open question that shows the patient has been heard. Focusing is the agreement on a topic. In pharmacy the topic is usually already set by the prescription, yet the pharmacist can still ask permission to discuss adherence or concerns. Evoking is the drawing out of the patient's own motivations. Planning is the collaborative development of a next step. In brief encounters planning is often a single, patient-owned action rather than a detailed written plan.

The processes are not rigid stages. A skilled pharmacist moves among them according to the patient's responses. The value of naming them is that they prevent the conversation from collapsing into pure information delivery.

4.3 A Practical Sequence for Two to Five Minutes

A workable sequence for most adherence conversations looks like this:

1. Brief engage: one reflection or open question that acknowledges the patient's opening statement or the situation (late refill, new start, expressed concern).
2. Permission and focus: "Would it be all right if we took a minute to look at how this is fitting with your routine?" or simply "Can I ask about the gap in refills?"
3. Evoke: one or two open questions or reflections aimed at the patient's own reasons, concerns, or previous efforts.
4. Offer information with permission if needed, then return the floor to the patient for interpretation.
5. Short summary and collaborative next step: "What do you want to try between now and the next fill?"

The entire sequence can be completed in under four minutes when the pharmacist stays disciplined. Each step uses the OARS skills from the previous chapter. The structure prevents the righting reflex from taking over at the first sign of hesitation.

4.4 Using Scaling Questions Efficiently

The readiness ruler is a simple scaling question that fits the brief format. “On a scale from 0 to 10, how ready do you feel to take this every day as prescribed?” Follow-up questions elicit change talk: “Why a 6 and not a 3?” or “What would it take to move from a 6 to a 7?” The numbers themselves are less important than the language the patient produces while explaining them.

Scaling questions work because they assume some readiness already exists and invite the patient to articulate it. They also avoid the binary trap of “Are you going to take it or not?” A patient who answers 4 is still offering information that can be explored. A patient who answers 8 can be asked what makes it an 8, thereby strengthening existing motivation.

In practice the ruler takes thirty to forty-five seconds and often yields more usable change talk than several minutes of advice.

4.5 Handling the Transition to Information

Pharmacists possess expertise that patients need. The structure does not eliminate information giving. It changes the timing and the framing. After the patient has been heard and has voiced some of their own thinking, the pharmacist asks permission: “Would it be helpful if I shared what we usually see with this side effect?” or “Can I give you one piece of information that addresses the concern you just raised?”

Permission does two things. It respects autonomy and it increases the likelihood that the patient will actually listen. After the information is given, the floor returns to the patient: “How does that land for you?” or “What do you make of that?” The patient’s interpretation, not the pharmacist’s delivery, determines whether the information will influence behavior.

4.6 Worked Example with Hollis

Hollis, a 71-year-old patient, is late on a refill of apixaban. The pharmacist, Indigo, has a short window.

Indigo: "I see the refill is about twelve days past due. What's been going on with taking it?" (engage and open question)

Hollis: "I ran out and kept forgetting to call. I feel fine."

Indigo: "You ran out, the call slipped, and since you're feeling okay it didn't feel urgent." (reflection)

Hollis: "Right."

Indigo: "On a scale of 0 to 10, how important is it to you to stay on this one steadily?" (scaling)

Hollis: "Maybe a 7. I know it's for the afib."

Indigo: "A 7. What makes it a 7 rather than a 4?" (evoking change talk)

Hollis: "I don't want a stroke. My neighbor had one."

Indigo: "You have a clear reason for staying consistent, and the running out got in the way. Would it be all right if I shared a couple of options that make the refills more automatic?" (permission)

After a brief exchange about 90-day supplies and pharmacy automatic refill, Indigo summarizes: "So the stroke risk is real for you, and setting up the automatic refill would take the remembering out of it. Does that feel like a workable next step?"

The conversation stays inside four minutes. Hollis has voiced a personal reason for adherence and left with a concrete, self-endorsed plan.

4.7 When the Structure Needs to Flex

Not every encounter follows the sequence cleanly. A patient in acute distress may need immediate practical help before any exploration of motivation. A patient who opens with strong change talk can move quickly to planning. A patient who is openly hostile may require more engaging and less focusing. The structure is a guide, not a rigid protocol. The pharmacist's judgment remains essential.

The most common reason the structure fails is the pharmacist's own anxiety about time or about losing control of the conversation. Practice reduces that anxiety. Once the sequence feels familiar, it actually saves time by preventing circular arguments and repeated unsuccessful advice giving.

What to Carry Forward

Unstructured informational counseling is efficient for data transfer and inefficient for behavior change. The four processes of engaging, focusing, evoking, and planning can be compressed into the pharmacy time window when the pharmacist selects moves deliberately. A practical five-part sequence keeps the conversation collaborative without extending it. Scaling questions rapidly elicit change talk. Information is offered with permission and then returned to the patient for interpretation. The worked encounter with Hollis shows the structure operating inside four minutes. Flexibility remains necessary, yet the default structure protects the conversation from collapsing into the righting reflex. The next chapter supplies ready language for the most common adherence situations pharmacists face.

Chapter 5.0: Everyday Adherence Scripts

A script is not a straitjacket. It is a starting set of words that already embody the spirit and the OARS skills so the pharmacist does not have to invent them under pressure. Once the underlying stance is solid, the words can be adapted freely.

5.1 Principles Behind the Scripts

Every script in this chapter follows the same logic. It begins with engagement rather than correction. It uses reflection before advice. It asks permission before offering information. It ends with a patient-owned next step or an open door for the next encounter. The language is deliberately plain and short enough for a noisy counter.

The scripts are written for common situations: new prescriptions, late refills, expressed side-effect concerns, cost barriers, and "I feel fine so I stopped." They are not exhaustive. They are models that can be modified for tone, regional speech, and individual patient language.

5.2 New Prescription Conversations

Patient presents a new chronic medication.

Pharmacist: "This is a new one for you. What have you already heard about it?"

(Patient responds.)

Pharmacist: "So you're coming in with [reflection of patient's knowledge or concern]. Would it be all right if I filled in a couple of the practical pieces and then we can see how it fits?"

After brief information: “What feels most important for you to remember about starting this?”

The opening open question surfaces existing knowledge and concerns immediately. The permission request keeps the pharmacist from launching into a monologue. The final question places ownership of the key points with the patient.

5.3 Late Refill or Gap in Therapy

Pharmacist: “I notice it’s been a bit longer than usual since the last fill. What’s been getting in the way?”

(Patient responds with forgetfulness, side effects, cost, or feeling well.)

Pharmacist: “That’s [reflection]. On a scale of 0 to 10, how important is it to you to stay on top of this one?”

(After answer): “What makes it that number and not a lower one?”

Then, if appropriate: “Would it help to look at one or two ways to make the refills easier?”

This sequence replaces the common “You need to take this every day” with exploration. The scaling question reliably produces change talk when any motivation exists.

5.4 Side Effect Concerns

Patient: “I think this is what’s making me [symptom].”

Pharmacist: “You’re connecting the [symptom] to the medicine and it’s bothering you.”

(Patient elaborates.)

Pharmacist: "That sounds disruptive. Would it be useful if I shared what we usually see with this side effect and the options for managing it?"

After information: "How does that information sit with you? What would you like to do next?"

The reflection prevents the immediate defensive correction ("It's probably not the medicine"). Permission keeps the information from feeling imposed. The final question returns decision making to the patient.

5.5 Cost Barriers

Patient expresses inability to afford the medication.

Pharmacist: "The cost is a real obstacle right now."

(Patient confirms.)

Pharmacist: "You still want the treatment if we can make the price workable. Would it be all right if I checked a couple of options—manufacturer programs, alternative drugs, or pharmacy discount routes—and we see what turns up?"

This script acknowledges the legitimacy of the barrier without treating it as the patient's failure. It moves quickly to collaborative problem solving while preserving autonomy.

5.6 "I Feel Fine So I Stopped"

Pharmacist: "You're feeling well and that makes the medicine feel less necessary."

(Patient agrees.)

Pharmacist: "A lot of people reach that point. What do you already know about what the medicine is doing in the background even when you feel okay?"

(After response, with permission if needed): "Would it help to look at what the numbers or the risks tend to do when the medicine is stopped for a while?"

Then: "Given that, where does that leave you about continuing?"

The script treats the "feeling fine" logic as understandable rather than irrational. It invites the patient to examine the asymptomatic nature of the condition without lecture.

5.7 Braided Cases of Script Use

Two short parallel cases illustrate adaptation.

Joss, age 52, late on a statin. The pharmacist uses the late-refill script, hears "I feel fine," shifts into the "feel fine" language, and ends with Joss agreeing to a 90-day supply and a reminder call. The encounter lasts three and a half minutes.

Kestrel, age 67, new start on an SGLT2 inhibitor. The pharmacist opens with the new-prescription question, hears concern about genital infections, reflects it, asks permission, provides prevention information, and closes with Kestrel stating the hygiene step they will take. Time: just under four minutes.

In both cases the pharmacist stayed inside the structure while adjusting the exact words to the patient's language. Neither encounter required a private counseling room.

5.8 Adapting Scripts to Personal Voice

Scripts fail when they sound recited. The pharmacist must adjust vocabulary, pace, and formality to match their own natural speech and the patient's. A formal "Would it be all right if I shared..." can become "Can I give you a quick piece of info on that?" without losing the permission element. A reflection can be shortened to a few words when the environment is noisy.

The discipline is to keep the underlying moves: engage first, reflect before advising, ask permission, return the floor. The surface language can vary widely.

5.9 When Scripts Are Not Enough

Some encounters exceed the capacity of a brief script. Severe distress, complex polypharmacy requiring reconciliation, or clear need for a longer clinical service should be escalated. The scripts are tools for the high-volume, high-frequency conversations that constitute most pharmacy counseling. They are not a substitute for comprehensive medication management when that service is indicated and available.

From Theory to Practice

The scripts operationalize the spirit and the OARS skills for the situations pharmacists encounter most often. New prescription, late refill, side-effect concern, cost barrier, and asymptomatic discontinuation each receive a short, adaptable sequence that begins with engagement and ends with patient ownership. Two parallel cases show the scripts functioning inside ordinary time limits. Adaptation to personal voice keeps the language natural. Escalation remains available when the brief format is insufficient. With these starting words in place, the pharmacist can focus attention on listening rather than on inventing the next sentence under pressure.

Chapter 6.0: Handling Ambivalence and Resistance

A patient says, "I know the numbers are high, but I feel fine and the medicine makes me tired." Two true statements sit side by side. One points toward action. The other points toward continuing as is. The pharmacist who treats the second statement as an obstacle to be removed usually strengthens it. The pharmacist who treats both statements as data usually learns something useful.

6.1 The Nature of Ambivalence

Ambivalence is the simultaneous presence of conflicting motivations. It is not a character flaw or a lack of education. It is the normal psychological state that precedes most sustained behavior change. Patients who appear purely resistant are often highly ambivalent; the sustain-talk side has simply become louder in the moment.

Miller and Rollnick observed that arguing for change when the patient is arguing for the status quo places the patient in the position of defending the status quo (Miller & Rollnick, 2013). The more the clinician pushes, the more the patient digs in. This is the opposite of the desired effect. The practical implication for pharmacy is immediate. When a patient voices hesitation, the first clinical task is to understand the hesitation accurately rather than to overpower it with additional facts.

Sustain talk is language that favors the status quo. Change talk is language that favors the desired behavior. Both appear in nearly every adherence conversation. The pharmacist's job is not to eliminate sustain talk. The job is to explore both sides with equal curiosity so that the patient's own change talk can grow louder.

6.2 Rolling with Resistance

Rolling with resistance means responding to sustain talk or discord without confrontation (Miller & Rollnick, 2013). The skill is primarily reflective. When a patient says, "I don't think I need this," a reflective response might be, "You're not convinced this is necessary for you right now." The reflection shows that the statement has been heard. It does not concede the clinical point. It simply removes the need for the patient to keep repeating or escalating the statement.

Two common reflective techniques are useful here. A simple reflection stays close to the words. A double-sided reflection acknowledges both sides of the ambivalence when both have been expressed: "On one hand the tiredness is a real problem, and on the other hand you want to keep your blood pressure from causing bigger issues." The double-sided form is especially effective because it places the conflict inside the patient rather than between patient and pharmacist.

Amplified reflection is a more advanced move. The pharmacist slightly overstates the sustain talk: "So this medicine is really not something you see any use for at all." Patients often respond by moderating their own statement, which produces change talk. The technique requires care. Overuse or inaccurate amplification can feel sarcastic. When it is delivered with genuine curiosity it frequently softens the position.

6.3 Discord Versus Sustain Talk

Discord is interpersonal. It appears as arguing, interrupting, discounting, or withdrawing from the relationship with the clinician. Sustain talk is intrapersonal. It is the patient's own arguments for not changing. The distinction matters because the responses differ. Discord often signals that the pharmacist has moved too far into the expert or directing role. The remedy is to return to engaging: more reflection, more emphasis on autonomy, less persuasion. Sustain talk is material to be explored rather than a relational rupture to be repaired.

In pharmacy settings the two frequently blend. A patient who feels lectured may express sustain talk more forcefully and may also show discord. The pharmacist who responds only to the content and ignores the relational signal often worsens both. A brief return to partnership language ("You're the one who has to live with this decision") can lower the temperature enough for exploration to continue.

6.4 Evoking Change Talk Without Pressure

Once sustain talk has been reflected and the relationship is stable, the pharmacist can invite change talk more directly. Questions that ask for elaboration on any existing change language are efficient. If the patient has said, "I know I should," a useful follow-up is, "What makes you say you should?" If the patient has mentioned a family member's health event, "How did that affect your thinking about your own risk?" keeps the focus on the patient's values.

The readiness ruler remains one of the fastest methods. After the patient gives a number, the follow-up "Why that number and not a lower one?" almost always produces change talk. The question assumes some motivation already exists and asks the patient to articulate it. Even a low number yields useful information and keeps the conversation collaborative.

6.5 Worked Example with Linden

Linden, age 59, presents for a refill of an antihypertensive that is seventeen days late. The profile shows consistent gaps over the past year.

Pharmacist: "I see the fills have been running behind for a while. What's been the hardest part about keeping it steady?"

Linden: "I forget when I feel okay. And it makes me a little dizzy sometimes if I take it early."

Pharmacist: “Feeling okay makes it easy to skip, and the dizziness is another reason to hesitate.” (double-sided reflection)

Linden: “Yeah. I don’t want to fall or something.”

Pharmacist: “The dizziness feels like a safety issue. On a scale of 0 to 10, how important is it to you to keep your pressure controlled?”

Linden: “About a 6.”

Pharmacist: “A 6. What makes it a 6 rather than a 3?”

Linden: “My father had a stroke. I don’t want that.”

Pharmacist: “You have a clear personal reason, and the side effect and the forgetting keep getting in the way. Would it be all right if we looked at one or two practical adjustments that might reduce the dizziness and make the daily dose easier to remember?”

The sustain talk was reflected rather than challenged. The change talk about the father was elicited and strengthened. Information and problem-solving were offered only after permission and after the patient’s own motivation had been voiced. The encounter remained brief.

6.6 When Resistance Persists

Some patients remain firmly in sustain talk despite skillful reflection. The pharmacist’s task at that point is to protect the relationship and leave the door open. A useful closing is, “It sounds like this is not the right time for a change. If things shift or you want to talk about options later, I’m here.” This statement honors autonomy, avoids power struggles, and keeps future conversations possible. Pressing further in the moment usually produces only more discord.

Documentation can note the discussion and the patient's current position without judgment. The next fill then becomes another opportunity rather than a continuation of an argument.

6.7 Building Comfort with Ambivalence

Pharmacists are trained to resolve problems. Ambivalence feels like an unresolved problem. The shift required by motivational interviewing is to treat ambivalence as the ordinary starting point rather than as a failure of counseling. Comfort with the patient's mixed feelings reduces the pharmacist's own anxiety and makes rolling with resistance more natural. Practice with colleagues or recorded role-plays accelerates the shift. Hearing oneself respond to sustain talk with reflection instead of correction builds the new habit.

Closing the Loop

Ambivalence is the normal presence of both sustain talk and change talk. Resistance and discord are signals to adjust the relational stance rather than to push harder. Rolling with resistance relies primarily on accurate reflection, including double-sided and carefully used amplified forms. Change talk is evoked by exploring the patient's own reasons and by simple scaling questions. The worked encounter with Linden shows the sequence operating inside ordinary pharmacy time. When resistance remains firm, protecting the relationship and leaving an open door is more effective than continued persuasion. Comfort with ambivalence itself is a clinical skill that develops with deliberate practice. The next chapter applies these same principles to conversations that carry higher emotional and clinical stakes.

Chapter 7.0: High-Stakes Conversations

Vaccine hesitancy, new injectable therapies for diabetes and weight, and opioid-related discussions share a common feature. The patient's concerns are often intense, the clinical stakes are high, and traditional persuasion frequently backfires. The same spirit and skills used for everyday adherence still apply. The emotional temperature simply requires more deliberate engaging and more careful pacing.

7.1 Shared Features of High Stakes Topics

These conversations activate stronger sustain talk and greater risk of discord. Patients may arrive with information from social networks, prior adverse experiences, or deep-seated beliefs about bodily autonomy. The pharmacist who opens with corrective facts often finds the patient more entrenched at the end of the exchange than at the beginning. The corrective impulse is understandable. The data on vaccine-preventable disease, on the benefits of GLP-1 agents when tolerated, and on the risks of opioid misuse are clear. Delivery of those data without first establishing partnership and acceptance commonly produces the opposite of the intended effect.

The structure remains the same: engage, seek permission to explore, reflect both sides, evoke the patient's own concerns and values, then offer information inside that relational frame. The difference is that engaging may take a larger share of the brief time available, and the pharmacist must tolerate more intense emotion without becoming defensive.

7.2 Vaccine Conversations

A patient declines or hesitates. The pharmacist's opening reflection of the hesitation itself often lowers intensity. "You're not sure this is right for you right now." Follow-up open questions explore the specific concern: safety, efficacy, timing, prior reactions, or distrust. Once the concern is clear, permission is requested before any data are offered. After the data, the floor returns to the patient: "How does that information fit with your concern?"

The goal is not immediate acceptance. The goal is a respectful exchange that leaves the patient more informed and the relationship intact. Many patients who leave without accepting the vaccine on that day return later. The earlier conversation that avoided argument makes the return possible.

Research and practice reports consistently show that motivational interviewing approaches increase vaccine acceptance compared with standard informational or persuasive styles, particularly among patients who begin the conversation hesitant rather than firmly opposed (Gagneur, 2020).

7.3 GLP-1 and Similar Injectable Therapies

These agents produce substantial clinical benefit for many patients and also produce gastrointestinal side effects that lead to early discontinuation. Patients often arrive already worried about nausea, vomiting, or the need for long-term use. A useful opening is to ask what the patient has already heard or what concerns them most. Reflection of those concerns, followed by realistic expectation-setting offered with permission, reduces the chance that the first side effect will feel like a betrayal of the counseling.

Persistence conversations follow the same pattern. When a patient reports early side effects and wants to stop, the pharmacist reflects the difficulty, explores what the patient was hoping the medicine would achieve, and only then discusses titration, dietary adjustments, or alternatives. The patient's original goals become the reference point rather than the pharmacist's preference for continuation.

7.4 Opioid Related Discussions

Conversations about opioid safety, tapering, or potential misuse require particular attention to stigma and discord. Patients may fear judgment, loss of pain control, or being labeled. Engaging language that separates the person from the risk is essential. Reflections that acknowledge the reality of pain and the legitimacy of concern about function reduce defensiveness.

When the clinical task is to discuss risk or to explore readiness for a change in regimen, scaling questions and careful evocation of the patient's own priorities (function, safety, family, work) keep the conversation collaborative. Information about overdose risk, naloxone, or tapering schedules is offered with permission and framed as support for the patient's stated goals rather than as a restriction imposed by the pharmacist.

7.5 Worked Example with Merritt

Merritt, age 34, declines a recommended vaccine during a routine pickup.

Pharmacist: "You're deciding to pass on it today."

Merritt: "I just don't trust them. I know people who had problems."

Pharmacist: "You've heard about people who had problems, and that makes you cautious." (reflection)

Merritt: "Yeah. I'd rather take my chances."

Pharmacist: "Taking your chances feels safer than taking the vaccine right now. What kinds of problems are you most concerned about?"

After hearing the specific concern, the pharmacist asks permission to share the data relevant to that concern, provides it briefly, and asks Merritt what sense to make of it. Merritt still declines that day. The pharmacist ends with, "If you want to talk more another time or if anything changes, I'm here." The relationship remains usable.

7.6 Worked Example with Nyx

Nyx, age 48, returns two weeks after starting a GLP-1 agent and reports significant nausea.

Pharmacist: "The nausea has been harder than you expected."

Nyx: "I can't keep working like this. I want to stop."

Pharmacist: "It's interfering with work and stopping feels like the only option right now. What were you hoping this medicine would do for you when you started?"

Nyx mentions weight and blood sugar goals. The pharmacist reflects those goals, asks permission to discuss practical adjustments that often reduce early nausea, and explores whether a short trial of those adjustments feels acceptable. Nyx agrees to three more days with dietary changes and a follow-up call. The original motivations remain the anchor.

7.7 Maintaining the Relationship Across Encounters

High-stakes topics are rarely resolved in a single brief conversation. The pharmacist who prioritizes the long-term relationship over immediate conversion creates the conditions for later change. Documentation of the patient's concerns and the respectful tone of the exchange helps the next clinician continue productively. Team consistency matters. A technician or colleague who later uses confrontational language can undo the earlier work.

Where This Leaves Us

High-stakes conversations about vaccines, GLP-1 therapies, and opioids intensify both sustain talk and the risk of discord. The same spirit and micro-skills remain effective when engaging and reflection receive greater emphasis and when information is offered only inside a frame of partnership. Vaccine discussions benefit from exploring the specific concern before any data. GLP-1 persistence conversations stay anchored to the patient's original goals. Opioid-related talks require explicit attention to stigma and to the legitimacy of pain. Two worked encounters illustrate the approach under realistic time and emotional pressure. Protecting the relationship across multiple visits often matters more than winning any single exchange. The next chapter examines adaptations required by literacy, culture, caregivers, and the physical constraints of the pharmacy environment.

Chapter 8.0: Special Patient Situations

The basic skills do not change when the patient has limited health literacy, comes from a different cultural background, relies on a caregiver, or stands in a noisy open counseling area. The application of the skills does. Adjustments in language, pacing, and involvement of others keep the conversation collaborative rather than exclusionary.

8.1 Health Literacy and Plain Language

Low health literacy is common and often invisible. Patients may nod while understanding little. Motivational interviewing already favors plain language because reflections and open questions work best when they are simple. The additional discipline is to avoid medical terms unless the patient uses them first, to reflect in everyday words, and to check understanding without turning the check into a test.

Teach-back can be integrated gently (Ha Dinh et al., 2016). After key information is given with permission, the pharmacist might say, "Just so I make sure I was clear, how would you explain the timing of this dose to someone at home?" The request is framed as a check on the pharmacist's clarity rather than on the patient's intelligence. When the patient struggles, the pharmacist takes responsibility and simplifies further.

Reflections remain powerful. A patient who says, "The doctor said my sugar is high," can hear back, "Your sugar numbers are up and that has you concerned." The reflection uses the patient's own level of language and invites elaboration.

8.2 Cultural Considerations

Culture shapes beliefs about medication, autonomy, family roles, and the meaning of illness. The pharmacist cannot know every cultural framework. The pharmacist can remain curious and avoid assuming that the clinical logic that makes sense to the pharmacist makes the same sense to the patient.

Open questions that invite the patient's perspective are the primary tool. "How does this medicine fit with how you usually take care of your health?" or "What do your family members think about starting this?" surface relevant beliefs without requiring the pharmacist to guess. Reflections of those beliefs demonstrate respect. Information is then offered in relation to the patient's stated values rather than in opposition to them.

Autonomy support remains central. In some cultures decision-making is collective. Involving the relevant family member, with the patient's permission, can be more effective than insisting on individual decision-making. The spirit of partnership expands to include the decision-making unit the patient recognizes.

8.3 Working with Caregivers

Caregivers often accompany older adults, patients with cognitive impairment, or patients with complex regimens. The caregiver may be the person who actually manages the medicines. Engaging both the patient and the caregiver, while still centering the patient's preferences, requires deliberate attention.

A useful opening is to greet the patient first and then invite the caregiver's perspective with the patient's consent. Reflections can include both voices. When the caregiver dominates, a gentle return to the patient ("I want to make sure we're also hearing what matters to you") restores balance. When the patient defers entirely, the pharmacist can still seek the patient's assent to the plan that emerges.

Affirmations directed at the caregiver's efforts build alliance. "You've been keeping track of a complicated set of medicines" recognizes real work and reduces defensiveness if later adjustments are needed.

8.4 Privacy and Environmental Constraints

Many community pharmacies lack private counseling rooms. Conversations occur at an open counter with other patients nearby. The lack of privacy limits depth and may cause patients to withhold sensitive concerns. The pharmacist can still use the core skills while adapting to the setting.

Lowered voice, positioning that creates a partial visual barrier, and explicit acknowledgment of the environment help. "I know it's open out here. We can keep this brief and practical." Sensitive topics may need to be deferred to a phone follow-up or a scheduled clinical service. The brief counter exchange can still establish partnership and identify the need for a better setting.

Time pressure interacts with the environment. The structured brief sequence from earlier chapters becomes even more important when interruptions are frequent. A single accurate reflection and one open question can still change the tone of an encounter that must end quickly.

8.5 Worked Example with Oakley

Oakley, age 78, arrives with an adult daughter. The prescription is a new anticoagulant. Oakley's health literacy appears limited; the daughter answers most questions.

Pharmacist (to Oakley first): "This is a new blood thinner. What have you been told about it so far?"

Oakley looks at the daughter. The pharmacist waits. Oakley says, "It stops clots."

Pharmacist: "It helps prevent clots. What's your biggest question about starting it?"

Oakley: "Will I bleed?"

Pharmacist: "The bleeding risk is on your mind." (reflection) Then, to both: "Would it be all right if I explained how we watch for that and what to do if it happens?"

After plain-language information and a teach-back request directed first to Oakley, the pharmacist affirms the daughter's support and confirms a simple daily routine that both can state back. The patient remains the primary focus even though the caregiver is actively involved.

8.6 Worked Example with Pax

Pax, age 45, has limited English proficiency and relies on a telephone interpreter. The conversation is slower by necessity. The pharmacist uses shorter sentences, pauses for interpretation, and relies heavily on reflections of the interpreted statements. Open questions are kept simple. Permission is requested before any extended information. The structure still holds; only the pace changes. The interpreter becomes part of the collaborative process rather than a mere conduit.

8.7 Knowing When to Escalate

Special situations sometimes exceed the capacity of a brief counter conversation. Significant cognitive impairment, complex social needs, or high-risk medication changes may require referral to a longer clinical service, a social worker, or a language-concordant provider. The motivational interviewing stance remains useful in making that referral collaboratively rather than unilaterally. The patient or caregiver is involved in recognizing the need for more support and in choosing the next step.

The Takeaways That Matter

Limited health literacy calls for plain language, patient-level reflections, and gentle teach-back framed as a check on the pharmacist's clarity. Cultural difference is met with curiosity and with questions that surface the patient's own framework rather than with assumptions. Caregivers are engaged while the patient's voice remains central. Open counseling areas and noise require abbreviated yet still structured exchanges and occasional deferral of sensitive topics. Two worked encounters demonstrate the adjustments in practice. Escalation remains available when the brief format cannot meet the clinical need. The same spirit and skills scale across these situations when the pharmacist stays responsive to the person in front of them rather than to a rigid script.

Chapter 9.0: Involving Technicians and Students

Most adherence conversations begin before the pharmacist speaks. A technician notices a late refill flag, a student reviews the profile during a rotation, or a support staff member hears the patient mention side effects while waiting. When those early moments are ignored or handled inconsistently, the pharmacist inherits a colder start. When the whole team shares a basic collaborative language, the pharmacist inherits a warmer one.

9.1 The Limits of Solo Counseling

Pharmacy workflow distributes patient contact across multiple roles. Technicians process the majority of refill and intake interactions. Students on introductory and advanced practice experiences conduct supervised counseling and medication history taking. Pharmacists perform the final clinical check and the higher-stakes conversations. If only the pharmacist uses motivational interviewing skills, the majority of touchpoints remain informational or purely transactional. Patients receive mixed messages. Opportunities to surface concerns early are lost.

Time pressure makes the solo model even less sustainable. A pharmacist who must personally initiate every adherence discussion will inevitably skip some. A technician who can recognize a gap, offer a brief nonjudgmental opening, and hand off cleanly multiplies the number of productive conversations the pharmacist can complete.

Training gaps compound the problem. Many technicians receive little formal communication training beyond customer service scripts. Students often learn motivational interviewing concepts in isolation from the technical workflow they will actually enter.

The result is a team that wants better conversations yet lacks a shared practical method.

9.2 Core Principles for Team Use

Three principles keep team involvement coherent. First, every role stays inside its scope. Technicians and students do not diagnose or independently alter therapy. They engage, reflect, and surface information so the pharmacist can act. Second, the spirit remains consistent. Partnership, acceptance, and autonomy support are not reserved for the pharmacist. A technician who lectures or a student who interrogates undoes the relational work. Third, handoffs are explicit and warm. The patient should experience continuity rather than repetition or contradiction.

These principles allow simplified versions of the OARS skills to be taught and used safely by non-pharmacist team members. The full clinical decision-making stays with the pharmacist. The conversational climate becomes a team product.

9.3 Technician Opening Moves

Technicians already ask practical questions about allergies, address changes, and payment. Adding one or two collaborative moves requires little extra time. Useful openings include:

"I notice this one is a little past due. Has anything made it harder to keep on schedule?"

"How has this medicine been treating you since the last fill?"

"Any new concerns before I send this through to the pharmacist?"

These are open or mildly open questions that invite more than a yes or no. When the patient responds with a concern, the technician can offer a simple reflection ("The stomach upset has been an issue") and then hand off: "I'm going to have the pharmacist take a closer look at that with you."

Technicians should not push for commitment or provide clinical advice. Their role is to notice, invite, reflect briefly, and escalate. Even this limited use of engaging and reflecting changes the quality of the subsequent pharmacist conversation. The patient has already been heard once and is less likely to feel ambushed.

9.4 Student Participation on Rotations

Students need deliberate practice under realistic conditions. Shadowing alone produces limited skill. Structured opportunities to conduct portions of the conversation, followed by immediate feedback, accelerate learning. Preceptors can assign specific micro-skills for a given shift: today the student will open every counseling encounter with an open question and one reflection before any information is given. Tomorrow the focus shifts to permission-asking and summaries.

Role-play with the preceptor or with peers before live patient contact reduces anxiety. Recorded or observed encounters, when feasible and consented, allow precise feedback on the ratio of questions to reflections and on the presence or absence of the righting reflex. Students consistently report that the skills feel awkward until they have used them repeatedly with real patients. Early supervised practice shortens that awkward period.

Students also benefit from learning the technician-level openings. Understanding the full workflow helps them integrate motivational interviewing into ordinary dispensing rather than treating it as a special counseling event.

9.5 Creating Shared Language Across the Team

A short team huddle or standing agenda item can establish common phrases and escalation criteria. Agreement on a few standard reflections and open questions prevents patients from hearing contradictory styles. Agreement on what warrants an immediate pharmacist handoff (expressed side-effect concerns, repeated late refills, vaccine hesitancy, cost barriers that affect adherence) keeps the workflow efficient.

Written quick-reference cards or posted examples at the technician workstation support consistency without requiring long training sessions. The goal is not uniform scripts for every person. The goal is a shared understanding of the relational stance and a small set of reliable moves that any team member can use.

9.6 Worked Example with Rumi

Rumi works as a technician in a high-volume community pharmacy. A patient arrives for a refill of a GLP-1 agent that is eleven days late. Rumi sees the flag.

Rumi: "I notice this one's past the usual fill date. How has it been going with the weekly dose?"

Patient: "The nausea was bad the first couple of weeks so I skipped a few."

Rumi: "The nausea made it hard to stay on schedule." (simple reflection)

Patient: "Yeah."

Rumi: "I'm going to have the pharmacist talk with you about that before we finish this up. They can look at options with you."

The handoff is clean. The pharmacist inherits a patient who has already named the barrier and has been met with acceptance rather than correction. The subsequent conversation can move directly into exploration and collaborative problem-solving instead of spending the first minute overcoming defensiveness.

9.7 Worked Example with Solstice

Solstice is a student on an advanced pharmacy practice experience. The preceptor has asked Solstice to open the next three counseling encounters with an open question and at least one reflection before giving any information. A patient presents a new antihypertensive.

Solstice: "This is a new blood pressure medicine. What questions or concerns do you already have about it?"

Patient: "I worry about feeling tired. A friend of mine had that."

Solstice: "You're concerned about tiredness because of what your friend experienced."

Patient: "Right. I drive a lot for work."

Solstice then asks permission to share typical side-effect information and monitoring advice, involves the preceptor for any clinical nuances, and ends by asking the patient what feels most important to watch for in the first weeks. The preceptor later debriefs the ratio of listening to informing and the quality of the reflection. Solstice leaves the shift with concrete feedback rather than a general impression.

9.8 Barriers to Team Adoption

Three barriers appear repeatedly. The first is the belief that communication skills are soft and secondary to technical accuracy. Data on adherence, safety, and patient experience contradict that belief, yet the culture of many pharmacies still prioritizes speed and error-free dispensing above conversational quality. Leadership endorsement and simple metrics (for example, tracking how often late-refill flags trigger a brief collaborative opening) help shift the culture.

The second barrier is fear of slowing the workflow. In practice, a ten-second open question and reflection often prevent longer downstream arguments or repeated failed counseling attempts. Time invested early is frequently recovered later.

The third barrier is inconsistent training. One-time in-services fade. Short, repeated practice with feedback sustains the skills better than a single workshop. Pairing new technicians with a colleague who already uses the openings creates informal modeling that formal training alone cannot achieve.

9.9 Measuring Team Progress

Simple process measures are more useful than distant outcome measures at the start. How often do technicians flag and open late-refill conversations? How often do students begin with an open question? How frequently does the pharmacist inherit a patient who has already voiced a concern in a non-defensive way? These indicators are observable, improvable, and directly tied to the daily work. Clinical outcomes such as proportion of days covered can be examined later once the process is reliable.

The Working Knowledge

Adherence conversations are team events whether the team acknowledges it or not. Technicians can safely use brief open questions and reflections to surface concerns and hand off cleanly. Students need structured, supervised practice of specific micro-skills with immediate feedback. Shared language and clear escalation criteria keep the patient experience consistent. Two worked examples show the technician opening and the student performance under ordinary conditions. Barriers of culture, time fear, and inconsistent training are real yet addressable with leadership support and repeated short practice. Process measures focused on conversational behavior provide the fastest feedback loop. When the whole team contributes to a collaborative climate, the pharmacist's limited counseling time becomes more productive and less exhausting.

Chapter 10.0: Sustaining the Skills

Learning the skills is the shorter task. Keeping them alive across months of high-volume shifts is the longer one. Without deliberate maintenance the righting reflex returns, reflections become scarce, and the old informational script reasserts itself.

10.1 Why Skills Decay

Motivational interviewing skills are not automatic for most clinicians. They compete with deeply practiced habits formed in training and reinforced by time pressure. When the environment rewards speed and documentation volume, the collaborative moves require extra cognitive effort. Under fatigue or interruption that extra effort is the first thing to drop. Studies of training in motivational interviewing across health professions show that initial gains fade within months unless followed by coaching, feedback, or structured practice (Schwalbe et al., 2014). Pharmacy is not exempt from the pattern.

Decay is not a personal failing. It is the predictable result of an environment that does not automatically support the new behavior. The solution is to build small, repeatable maintenance structures into ordinary work rather than relying on permanent motivation.

10.2 Deliberate Practice in Ordinary Shifts

Deliberate practice focuses on a specific skill, includes immediate feedback, and occurs at a level that is challenging but achievable. In a pharmacy this can be as simple as choosing one micro-skill for a shift or a week. One week the focus is accurate simple reflections. The next week it is permission-asking before information. The following week it is ending with a patient-owned next step. The constraint keeps attention sharp and makes success observable.

A practical method is the end-of-shift note. In two minutes the pharmacist or student writes: What skill did I practice today? Where did it go well? Where did the old habit reappear? What will I try tomorrow? The note requires no special form. It creates a feedback loop that pure experience does not provide.

Peer observation, when feasible, accelerates improvement. Two colleagues agree to watch for a single skill during a shared shift or to debrief three encounters at the end of the day. The observation is specific and non-evaluative of overall performance. "I heard three reflections in that conversation" is more useful than "You did a good job."

10.3 Feedback That Improves Performance

Effective feedback is timely, specific, and focused on behavior rather than character. "You asked permission before giving the side-effect information" is usable. "You're a natural at this" is not. Students and technicians especially benefit from feedback that names the exact move that worked or the exact moment the righting reflex appeared.

Self-feedback through brief audio recording (with appropriate consent and privacy safeguards) remains one of the most powerful methods. Hearing oneself interrupt, advise without permission, or miss a clear piece of change talk is often more corrective than any external comment. Even one recorded encounter per month can reset drifting habits.

10.4 Building Environmental Supports

Individual willpower is a weak foundation. Environmental supports are stronger. Examples include:

A laminated card at the counseling window with three open questions and the readiness-ruler follow-ups.

A standing agenda item in team meetings: one recent adherence conversation that went well and one that did not, examined only for conversational process.

A shared electronic note template that prompts documentation of the patient's stated concern and the collaborative next step rather than only the information given.

Recognition of process behaviors (for example, noting when a technician consistently opens late-refill conversations) rather than only clinical outcomes.

These supports make the desired behavior easier and the old behavior slightly harder. Over time the collaborative approach becomes the path of least resistance.

10.5 Linking Skills to Professional Sustainability

Pharmacists who use motivational interviewing consistently often report lower frustration with nonadherence. The shift from "I failed to convince the patient" to "I offered a respectful opportunity for change" reduces the personal toll of repeated unsuccessful persuasion. Burnout literature in health care repeatedly identifies lack of control and repeated moral distress as contributors (Maslach & Leiter, 2016). A conversational method that restores a sense of skillful action inside constrained time addresses both factors.

The link is not automatic. It requires noticing the difference in one's own emotional state after collaborative versus directive encounters. That noticing itself becomes part of the maintenance practice.

10.6 Worked Example with Tatum

Tatum is a pharmacist three months out of an initial motivational interviewing workshop. Early enthusiasm has faded under volume pressure. Reflections have become rare. Tatum decides to reclaim one skill for two weeks: every counseling encounter will contain at least one accurate reflection before any advice. At the end of each shift Tatum notes the approximate percentage of encounters in which the goal was met and one example of a reflection that changed the tone. After ten shifts the percentage has risen from roughly 30 percent to over 80 percent. The righting reflex still appears, yet it is caught and corrected more often. Tatum reports that the conversations feel less combative and that the end-of-day fatigue is slightly lower.

10.7 Worked Example with Tierney

Tierney precepts students and wants the skills to survive beyond the rotation. Each student receives a single micro-skill focus for the first week and a different focus for the second. Daily two-minute debriefs address only that skill. Students leave with a written personal maintenance plan: one skill to practice for the first month of their next rotation or job, a method for self-feedback, and a request to their future preceptor or manager for occasional observation. Follow-up emails three months later show that students who left with a concrete plan report higher continued use than those who left with only general encouragement.

10.8 When Maintenance Fails

Even well-designed systems lapse during staffing shortages, personal stress, or leadership turnover. The response is the same as with a patient who has relapsed on a medication: treat the lapse as information rather than as proof of permanent failure. Re-start with a single skill, a short time horizon, and visible tracking. Shame prolongs the lapse. Curiosity shortens it.

Looking Back and Ahead

Skills decay under ordinary pharmacy conditions unless deliberate maintenance is built into the work. Single-skill focus for short periods, end-of-shift notes, specific peer or self-feedback, and environmental prompts form a practical maintenance system. Two examples show a pharmacist reclaiming a drifting skill and a preceptor equipping students for continued use. Linking the conversational method to reduced professional frustration strengthens motivation to sustain it. Lapses are expected and recoverable. The habits formed in daily brief encounters determine whether motivational interviewing remains a living practice or becomes a workshop memory. The final chapters integrate these skills into a coherent professional stance and point toward continued growth.

Chapter 11.0: Measuring Outcomes and Growth

Two pharmacists leave the same shift. Both spoke with patients about late refills and new starts. One feels drained and uncertain whether any of it mattered. The other feels tired yet clear about what went well and what to adjust tomorrow. The difference is rarely the patients. It is whether the pharmacist has a practical way to notice process and progress.

11.1 The Problem of Invisible Results

Adherence outcomes move slowly. Proportion of days covered, persistence curves, and A1C or blood pressure changes appear weeks or months later. A single counseling encounter rarely produces a visible clinical shift by the next morning. When pharmacists judge their effectiveness only by immediate patient agreement or by distant quality metrics, they receive almost no usable feedback. The absence of feedback invites either unjustified optimism or quiet demoralization.

Quality metrics such as Medicare Star Ratings reward improvements in adherence for specific drug classes (Spears et al., 2020). Those metrics are real and financially consequential for many organizations. They are also lagging and noisy. They cannot tell a pharmacist whether today's three-minute conversation was skillful. Relying on them alone leaves the daily work unguided.

Process measures solve the visibility problem. They track the conversational behaviors the pharmacist can control: whether an open question was asked, whether a reflection preceded advice, whether permission was requested before information, whether the patient voiced any change talk, whether a collaborative next step was stated. These indicators are observable in real time. They improve with practice. They form the bridge between the skills taught in earlier chapters and any later clinical or quality outcome.

11.2 Process Measures That Fit Pharmacy Work

Useful process measures are few, concrete, and countable. Examples include:

- Percentage of counseling encounters that began with an open question or a reflection rather than with unsolicited information.
- Number of times permission was asked before clinical advice or data were given.
- Presence or absence of at least one patient statement that qualifies as change talk.
- Whether the encounter ended with a next step the patient themselves endorsed.

A pharmacist can track one or two of these for a week using simple tally marks on a scrap of paper or a quick electronic note. The act of tracking itself sharpens attention. What gets counted gets noticed. What gets noticed becomes easier to improve.

Team-level process measures extend the same logic. How often do technicians open a late-refill conversation with a nonjudgmental question? How often does a student hand off a patient who has already named a concern? These counts reveal whether the collaborative climate is spreading or remaining isolated to one or two individuals.

11.3 Linking Process to Intermediate Outcomes

Process measures gain power when they are occasionally linked to intermediate outcomes the pharmacy can see. Refill timing for patients who received a collaborative conversation versus those who received only standard counseling can be compared over a month. Vaccine acceptance rates after motivational interviewing-style discussions can be examined against baseline. Early discontinuation rates for GLP-1 agents after realistic expectation-setting conversations can be tracked.

These comparisons are not formal research. They are practical learning tools. Even imperfect local data help a pharmacist or a team see whether the conversational investment is associated with movement in the desired direction. When the association appears, motivation to sustain the skills increases. When it does not, the team can examine fidelity: were the skills actually used, or was the old script simply relabeled?

11.4 Personal Growth Metrics

Professional growth requires a second set of indicators focused on the clinician rather than the patient. Useful questions include:

- How often did I catch myself in the righting reflex and correct course?
- How frequently did I leave an encounter feeling that the patient had been heard?
- Did my frustration with nonadherence decrease, increase, or stay the same this week?
- What specific skill feels more automatic than it did last month?

These questions can be answered in a two-minute end-of-week note. Over months they reveal trajectory. Pharmacists who track only patient outcomes often miss their own increasing fluency and decreasing emotional toll. Pharmacists who track both stay oriented to the dual purpose of the work: better patient care and sustainable professional practice.

11.5 Worked Example with Umber

Umber is a clinical pharmacist responsible for a panel of patients with diabetes and cardiovascular risk. After six weeks of deliberate focus on reflections and permission-asking, Umber begins a simple tracking sheet. Each counseling note includes two checkboxes: “Opened with open question or reflection” and “Patient voiced change talk.” At the end of the first month the open-question rate sits at 70 percent and change-talk presence at 45 percent. Umber also notes personal frustration on a 0-to-10 scale at the end of each week. The frustration score trends downward even though several patients remain nonadherent. The process data show skill use. The personal data show reduced emotional cost. Both support continued effort.

11.6 Worked Example with Vesper

Vesper manages a community pharmacy team. The team agrees to track one process measure for technicians: late-refill flags that receive a brief collaborative opening before pharmacist involvement. Baseline is near zero. After two weeks of coaching and a simple reminder card, the rate rises to roughly half of eligible flags. Vesper reviews the numbers in a short team huddle, celebrates the increase, and asks for one barrier that still prevents the other half. The discussion surfaces a workflow timing issue that is then adjusted. The metric remains visible on a shared board for the next month. Adherence numbers for the tracked drug class begin to show modest improvement several weeks later. The team can see the chain from conversational behavior to intermediate result.

11.7 Avoiding Common Measurement Traps

Three traps undermine measurement efforts. The first is tracking too many indicators at once. Attention fragments and the practice collapses. One or two process measures are sufficient to start. The second is treating process measures as performance judgment rather than as learning data. When counts become tied to formal evaluation without adequate support, gaming and resentment appear. The third is expecting immediate clinical outcome shifts. Process change precedes outcome change.

Demanding instant Star Ratings movement from a new conversational habit sets the effort up for apparent failure.

Measurement works best when it is owned by the people doing the work, kept light, and used for adjustment rather than for blame.

11.8 Integrating Measurement into Ordinary Routine

The most sustainable systems require almost no extra time. A single checkbox in an existing electronic note, a tally on a daily worksheet already in use, or a two-minute standing item in a team huddle can carry the practice. Formal dashboards and lengthy reports are unnecessary at the beginning and often counterproductive. Complexity kills maintenance. Simplicity sustains it.

Students can be given a personal process card for a rotation. Technicians can track openings for a defined period and then discuss the experience. Pharmacists can choose a quarterly personal skill audit. The exact form matters less than the presence of some regular, low-burden feedback loop.

What We Now Know

Distant adherence metrics and quality ratings matter organizationally yet provide almost no daily guidance to the pharmacist. Process measures focused on conversational behavior make skill use visible and improvable in real time. Intermediate outcomes such as refill timing or early discontinuation rates can be examined locally to test whether the process investment is associated with movement. Personal growth metrics track fluency and emotional sustainability alongside patient indicators. Two examples show an individual pharmacist and a team using light tracking to guide effort and observe progress. Common traps of over-measurement, punitive use, and impatience with lagging outcomes are avoidable. The lightest systems that produce regular feedback are the ones that survive contact with ordinary pharmacy work. Measurement, kept simple and learning-oriented, closes the loop between the skills developed in this book and the ongoing professional practice that keeps them alive.

Conclusion: From Counter Conversations to Lasting Partnership

The work of this book began with a number large enough to demand attention and ended with the smallest practical unit of professional behavior: one open question, one reflection, one moment of permission, one patient-owned next step. Between those poles lies a coherent method for turning the ordinary pharmacy encounter into an opportunity for genuine partnership.

Nonadherence remains costly in human and economic terms. Traditional informational counseling, however well-intentioned, frequently activates resistance rather than motivation. The spirit of motivational interviewing—partnership, acceptance, compassion, and evocation—reorients the pharmacist from expert persuader to collaborative guide. The OARS micro-skills translate that spirit into words that fit the two-to-five-minute window. A simple structure keeps the conversation from collapsing into advice-giving under pressure. Ready language for common situations reduces the cognitive load of inventing every sentence in the moment. The same principles scale to high-stakes topics, to patients with limited literacy or different cultural frames, and to the realities of open counseling areas and caregiver involvement.

None of this work stays alive if it remains the possession of a single motivated pharmacist. Technicians can open conversations and hand off cleanly. Students can practice specific skills under supervision and carry maintenance plans into their next setting. Teams that share a short list of collaborative moves create a consistent patient experience and multiply the pharmacist's limited counseling time. Skills decay without deliberate maintenance; single-skill focus, brief feedback, and light environmental supports keep them usable across months and years. Process measures make the daily work visible so that growth can be noticed and adjusted in real time.

The method does not guarantee adherence. Patients retain autonomy, including the autonomy to decline. What the method does guarantee is that the pharmacist has offered a respectful, skillful opportunity for the patient to hear their own reasons for change. That stance reduces the moral distress of repeated unsuccessful persuasion and restores a sense of professional effectiveness inside constrained time. Over repeated encounters the cumulative effect on adherence, on trust, and on the pharmacist's own sustainability becomes measurable.

The counter remains crowded. The next patient is already waiting. The invitation of this book is to meet that patient with one different move—an open question instead of an assumption, a reflection instead of a correction, a moment of permission instead of an immediate lecture—and to notice what becomes possible. Partnership is not a destination. It is a way of conducting the next conversation, and the one after that.

Bonus Resources and Appendices

These resources are designed for immediate use at the counter, in team huddles, during precepting, or for personal practice. They distill the core methods from the preceding chapters into portable, low-burden tools. Photocopy, laminate, or adapt them to your local workflow and electronic systems.

Appendix A: Quick-Reference OARS and Conversation Structure Card

OARS at a Glance

- **Open questions**: Invite the patient's perspective. Examples: "What has been getting in the way?" "How are you feeling about starting this?" "What do you already know about it?"
- **Affirmations**: Notice real effort or strength. Examples: "You made it in today despite the schedule." "You've been consistent with the other medicines."
- **Reflections**: Return the patient's meaning. Simple: "The tiredness is bothering you." Complex: "The tiredness is making you wonder whether it's worth continuing."
- **Summaries**: Gather key points and transition. Example: "So the side effect is disruptive, and you still want the blood pressure controlled. Where does that leave you?"

Brief Conversation Structure (2–5 minutes)

1. Engage with one open question or reflection.
2. Ask permission to explore or share information.
3. Evoke with scaling, open questions, or reflections of change talk.
4. Offer information only with permission, then return the floor.

5. Close with a short summary and a patient-owned next step (or an open door).

Keep this card at the counseling window or in a pocket. One accurate move from the card is more useful than a perfect theoretical sequence left unused.

Appendix B: Script Library by Common Scenario

New Prescription "This is a new one for you. What have you already heard about it?" (Reflect response.) "Would it be all right if I filled in a couple of practical points and then we see how it fits for you?" (After information.) "What feels most important for you to remember as you start?"

Late Refill or Gap "I notice it's been longer than usual between fills. What's been getting in the way?" (Reflect.) "On a scale of 0 to 10, how important is it to you to stay on top of this one?" "What makes it that number and not a lower one?" "Would it help to look at one or two ways to make the refills easier?"

Side-Effect Concern "You're connecting [symptom] to the medicine and it's a problem." (Reflect further if needed.) "Would it be useful if I shared what we usually see with this and the options for managing it?" (After information.) "How does that sit with you? What would you like to do next?"

Cost Barrier "The cost is a real obstacle right now." "You still want the treatment if we can make the price workable. Would it be all right if I checked a couple of options and we see what turns up?"

"I Feel Fine So I Stopped" "You're feeling well and that makes the medicine feel less necessary." "What do you already know about what the medicine is doing in the background even when you feel okay?" (With permission if needed.) "Would it help to look at what tends to happen to the numbers or the risks when it's stopped for a while?" "Given that, where does that leave you about continuing?"

Adapt the exact wording to your natural speech and the patient's language. Preserve the sequence: engage, reflect, permission, patient interpretation, collaborative close.

Appendix C: Readiness Ruler and Change-Talk Cue Sheet

Readiness Ruler "On a scale from 0 to 10, how ready do you feel to [take this every day / stay on this / get the vaccine]?"

Follow-ups that elicit change talk:

- "Why that number and not a lower one?"
- "What would it take to move up one point?"
- "What makes it as high as it is?"

Change-Talk Cues to Listen For and Reflect Desire: "I want…" "I wish…" "I hope…" Ability: "I could…" "I can…" "I might be able to…" Reasons: "I would feel better if…" "It matters because…" Need: "I have to…" "I need to…" "I should…" Commitment: "I will…" "I plan to…" "I'm going to…" Taking steps: "I already started…" "I've been trying…"

When you hear any of these, reflect them. "You want to avoid what happened to your father." Strengthening change talk is more efficient than arguing against sustain talk.

Appendix D: Technician Quick-Start Phrases

Technicians stay inside scope: notice, invite, reflect briefly, hand off.

- "I notice this one is a little past due. Has anything made it harder to keep on schedule?"
- "How has this medicine been treating you since the last fill?"
- "Any new concerns before I send this through to the pharmacist?"
- Simple reflection after a concern: "The [side effect / cost / schedule] has been an issue."
- Warm handoff: "I'm going to have the pharmacist take a closer look at that with you."

Escalate immediately for expressed side effects, repeated gaps, vaccine hesitancy, cost barriers affecting adherence, or any clinical uncertainty. Do not provide clinical advice or push for commitment.

Appendix E: Self- and Peer-Observation Checklist

Use after a shift, a recorded encounter (with consent), or a peer observation. Mark only what you observe. Focus on one or two items per session.

- Began with open question or reflection rather than unsolicited information.
- Asked permission before giving advice or data.
- Offered at least one accurate reflection of the patient's words or meaning.
- Affirmed a real effort or strength (specific, not generic).
- Heard and reflected any change talk.
- Ended with a next step the patient endorsed or an open door.
- Caught and corrected a righting-reflex moment.
- Stayed within ordinary time limits.

Peer version: Replace "I" with "the clinician" and share only the observed behaviors, not overall judgments. One specific observation is more useful than general praise or criticism.

Appendix F: Sample Documentation Language

Keep notes concise and focused on process plus plan. Examples:

- "Discussed late refill. Patient noted [barrier]. Reflected concern. Patient voiced [change talk]. Collaborative plan: [patient-owned step]."
- "New start counseling. Opened with patient's existing knowledge. Permission obtained before side-effect information. Patient identified [key point] to monitor. Follow-up as needed."
- "Vaccine discussion. Patient expressed [specific concern]. Concern reflected. Information offered with permission. Patient declined today; door left open for future discussion."
- "Technician flagged gap and patient concern re: [issue]. Pharmacist explored with OARS approach. Plan: [step]."

These phrasings support continuity, quality review, and MTM documentation without requiring lengthy narrative.

Appendix G: Further Learning and Practice Pointers

Continued growth rests on deliberate practice rather than additional theory alone. Options that align with the methods in this book include:

- Structured role-play with colleagues focused on one micro-skill at a time.
- Periodic self-recording of brief encounters (privacy and consent required) followed by review against the observation checklist.
- Team huddles that examine one recent conversation solely for process (what move helped, what righting-reflex moment appeared).
- Precepting assignments that give students a single skill focus per week with daily two-minute feedback.
- Organizational support for light process tracking (checkboxes, tallies, or shared boards) rather than complex new systems.

Formal continuing-education programs in motivational interviewing exist through professional organizations. Choose those that emphasize observed practice and feedback over lecture alone. The skills remain usable only when they are practiced inside the actual time and workflow constraints of pharmacy practice.

These appendices are starting tools. Adapt them, shorten them, or expand them to fit your setting. The measure of their value is whether they make the next conversation at the counter slightly more collaborative than the last.

References

Abughosh, S., Wang, X., Serna, O., Esse, T., Mann, A., Masilamani, S., Holstad, M. M., Essien, E. J., & Fleming, M. (2017). A motivational interviewing intervention by pharmacy students to improve medication adherence. *Journal of Managed Care & Specialty Pharmacy, 23*(5), 549–560. https://doi.org/10.18553/jmcp.2017.23.5.549

Amrhein, P. C., Miller, W. R., Yahne, C. E., Palmer, M., & Fulcher, L. (2003). Client commitment language during motivational interviewing predicts drug use outcomes. *Journal of Consulting and Clinical Psychology, 71*(5), 862–878. https://doi.org/10.1037/0022-006X.71.5.862

Berger, B. A., & Villaume, W. A. (2013). *Motivational interviewing for health care professionals: A sensible approach.* American Pharmacists Association.

Gagneur, A. (2020). Motivational interviewing: A powerful tool to address vaccine hesitancy. *Canada Communicable Disease Report, 46*(4), 93–97. https://doi.org/10.14745/ccdr.v46i04a06

Ha Dinh, T. T., Bonner, A., Clark, R., Ramsbotham, J., & Hines, S. (2016). The effectiveness of the teach-back method on adherence and self-management in health education for people with chronic disease: A systematic review. *JBI Database of Systematic Reviews and Implementation Reports, 14*(1), 210–247. https://doi.org/10.11124/jbisrir-2016-2296

Jalal, Z., Akhtar, S., Finlay, K., King, K., Goel, N., & Ward, J. (2019). Perceptions of UK community pharmacists on current consultation skills and motivational interviewing as a consultation approach: A qualitative study.

Pharmacy, 7(2), 52. https://doi.org/10.3390/pharmacy7020052

Kelling, S. E. (2015). Exploring accessibility of community pharmacy services. *INNOVATIONS in Pharmacy, 6*(3). https://doi.org/10.24926/iip.v6i3.392

Maslach, C., & Leiter, M. P. (2016). Understanding the burnout experience: Recent research and its implications for psychiatry. *World Psychiatry, 15*(2), 103–111. https://doi.org/10.1002/wps.20311

Miller, W. R. (1983). Motivational interviewing with problem drinkers. *Behavioural Psychotherapy, 11*(2), 147–172. https://doi.org/10.1017/S0141347300006583

Miller, W. R., & Rollnick, S. (2013). *Motivational interviewing: Helping people change* (3rd ed.). Guilford Press.

Schwalbe, C. S., Oh, H. Y., & Zweben, A. (2014). Sustaining motivational interviewing: A meta-analysis of training studies. *Addiction, 109*(8), 1287–1294. https://doi.org/10.1111/add.12558

Spears, J., Erkens, J., Misquitta, C., Cutler, T., & Stebbins, M. (2020). A pharmacist-led, patient-centered program incorporating motivational interviewing for behavior change to improve adherence rates and star ratings in a Medicare plan. *Journal of Managed Care & Specialty Pharmacy, 26*(1), 35–41. https://doi.org/10.18553/jmcp.2020.26.1.35

Watanabe, J. H., McInnis, T., & Hirsch, J. D. (2018). Cost of prescription drug–related morbidity and mortality. *Annals of Pharmacotherapy, 52*(9), 829–837. https://doi.org/10.1177/1060028018765159